THE KEYS TO LIVING YOUR LONGEST AND HEALTHIEST LIFE

Muhammad Rao

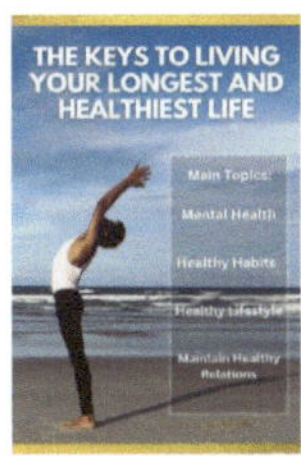

CONTENTS

MUHAMMAD RAO

The Keys to Living Your Longest and Healthiest Life

CHAPTER # 1

IMPORTANCE OF MENTAL HEALTH

Introduction

Mental health refers to the overall psychological, emotional, and social well-being of an individual. It affects how a person thinks, feels, and behaves in different situations. Health is a crucial aspect of an individual's life as it affects their ability to cope with daily stressors and maintain healthy relationships. We will discuss various aspects of health, including its definition, the importance of mental health, mental health disorders, factors affecting mental health, and ways to maintain good health.

Definition Of Mental Health

Mental health refers to the state of a person's mind and emotions. It encompasses the way an individual thinks, feels, and behaves in different situations. Mental health is a broad term that includes a range of psychological, emotional, and social factors that contribute to an individual's overall well-being. It is not just the absence of mental illness, but also the ability to cope with daily stressors and maintain healthy relationships.

1) Importance

Mental health is essential for an individual's overall well-being. It affects the way a person thinks, feels, and behaves in different situations. Good mental health is crucial for maintaining healthy relationships, coping with daily stressors, and achieving success in various aspects of life, including work, school, and personal life. It also contributes to physical health, as poor mental health can lead to various physical health problems, including heart disease, diabetes, and obesity.

2) Mental Health Disorders

Mental health disorders are conditions that affect an individual's mental health, emotions, and behavior. They can range from mild to severe and can impact an individual's ability to function in daily life. Mental health disorders can affect anyone, regardless of their age, gender, or social status. Some common mental health disorders include:

Anxiety disorders: Anxiety disorders are characterized by excessive worry and fear about everyday situations. They can include generalized anxiety disorder, panic disorder, social anxiety disorder, and specific phobias.

Mood disorders: Mood disorders are characterized by persistent feelings of sadness or hopelessness. They can include major depressive disorder, bipolar disorder, and seasonal affective disorder.

Personality disorders: Personality disorders are characterized by patterns of thoughts, feelings, and behaviors that deviate from societal norms. They can include borderline personality disorder, narcissistic personality disorder, and antisocial personality disorder.

Psychotic disorders: Psychotic disorders are characterized by a loss of touch with reality. They can include schizophrenia and delusional disorder.

Eating disorders: Eating disorders are characterized by abnormal eating habits that can lead to severe physical and mental health problems. They can include anorexia nervosa, bulimia nervosa, and binge-eating disorder.

3) Factors Affecting Mental Health

Several factors can affect an individual's mental health. Some of the common factors include:

Genetics: Genetics can play a role in the development of mental health disorders. Certain genes can make an individual more susceptible to mental health disorders.

Environment: The environment can also play a significant role in mental health. Exposure to stressors such as trauma, abuse, neglect, and poverty can increase the risk of mental health disorders.

Lifestyle factors: Lifestyle factors such as diet, exercise, sleep, and substance use can also affect mental health. A healthy lifestyle can help to promote good mental health.

Social factors: Social factors such as social support, relationships, and socioeconomic status can also affect mental health. Lack of social support and poor relationships can increase the risk of mental health disorders.

4) Ways to Maintain Good Mental Health

Maintaining good mental health is crucial for an individual's overall well-being. Here are some ways to maintain good mental health:

Practice self-care: Self-care involves taking care of oneself physically, emotionally, and mentally.

A healthy lifestyle is a way of living that promotes physical, mental, and emotional well-being. It is characterized by behaviors and habits that promote good health and reduce the risk of chronic diseases. A healthy lifestyle involves making informed decisions about diet, exercise, sleep, stress management, and other health-related behaviors. In this , we will discuss the importance of a healthy lifestyle, the components of a healthy lifestyle Maintaining good mental health is essential for overall well-being and quality of life. Good mental health involves feeling positive, coping with stress effectively, and being able to engage in daily activities without significant difficulties. In this , we will discuss several ways to maintain good mental health.

Prioritize self-care: Self-care involves taking care of oneself both physically and emotionally. This can include getting adequate sleep, exercising regularly, eating a healthy diet, and engaging in activities that promote relaxation and reduce stress.

Build and maintain relationships: Strong relationships with family, friends, and community members can provide social support and reduce the risk of mental health issues. Joining a social group or participating in community events can help to build and maintain these relationships.

Seek professional help: Seeking professional help can be crucial for maintaining good mental health. This can include therapy, counseling, or medication if necessary. Professional help can provide coping strategies, tools, and resources to manage mental health issues effectively.

Practice mindfulness: Mindfulness involves paying attention to the present moment and being aware of one's thoughts and emotions. It can help to reduce stress, improve mood, and increase self-awareness.

Stay active: Regular physical activity can improve mood, reduce stress, and increase self-esteem. Exercise can also help to improve cognitive function and reduce the risk of depression and anxiety.

Practice gratitude: Focusing on what one is grateful for can help to shift the focus away from negative thoughts and emotions. Practicing gratitude can help to increase positive emotions and improve overall well-being.

Limit social media use: Social media can be a significant source of stress and anxiety. Limiting social media use or taking breaks can help to reduce stress and improve overall mental health.

Get enough sleep: Adequate sleep is crucial for maintaining good mental health. Establishing a regular sleep schedule and creating a relaxing bedtime routine can help to improve sleep quality.

Manage stress: Stress can significantly impact mental health. Effective stress management techniques include exercise, meditation, deep breathing, or yoga. Identifying sources of stress and taking steps to minimize them can also help to manage stress effectively.

Engage in enjoyable activities: Engaging in activities that are enjoyable and bring a sense of purpose can help to improve overall mental health. This can include hobbies, volunteering, or spending time with loved ones.

In conclusion, maintaining good mental health is essential for overall well-being and quality of life. Prioritizing self-care, building and maintaining relationships, seeking professional help, practicing mindfulness, staying active, practicing gratitude, limiting social media use, getting enough sleep, managing stress, and engaging in enjoyable activities are all ways to maintain good mental health. It is important to recognize that mental health is just as important as physical health and to seek help if needed., and ways to achieve and maintain a healthy lifestyle.

CHAPTER # 2

IMPORTANCE OF A HEALTHY LIFESTYLE

A healthy lifestyle is essential for maintaining good health and preventing chronic diseases such as heart disease, diabetes, and cancer. It can also improve mental health, increase energy levels, and enhance overall well-being. A healthy lifestyle can help to reduce the risk of premature death and improve quality of life. It is never too late to adopt healthy habits, and small changes can make a big difference in overall health.

Components of a Healthy Lifestyle

A healthy lifestyle consists of several components, including:

Diet: A healthy diet includes a variety of fruits, vegetables, whole grains, lean protein, and healthy fats. It is low in saturated and trans fats, sodium, and added sugars. A healthy diet can reduce the risk of chronic diseases such as heart disease and diabetes.

Exercise: Regular physical activity can improve cardiovascular health, increase energy levels, and reduce the risk of chronic diseases. The American Heart Association recommends at least 150 minutes of moderate-intensity aerobic exercise per week.

Sleep: Getting adequate sleep is crucial for overall health and well-being. Adults should aim for 7-8 hours of sleep per night, while children and teenagers need more.

Stress management: Chronic stress can increase the risk of chronic diseases such as heart disease and depression. Effective stress management techniques include meditation, deep breathing, and exercise.

Substance use: Avoiding tobacco and excessive alcohol consumption can improve overall health and reduce the risk of chronic diseases.

Social connections: Social connections can improve mental health and reduce the risk of chronic diseases. Building and maintaining relationships with family and friends can promote overall well-being.

Ways to Achieve and Maintain a Healthy Lifestyle

Set realistic goals: Setting realistic goals can help to maintain motivation and prevent discouragement. Start with small goals and gradually increase the level of difficulty.

Seek support: Seek support from family, friends, or a healthcare provider. Joining a support group or seeking professional help can also provide accountability and motivation.

Keep a food diary: Keeping a food diary can help to identify areas for improvement in the diet. It can also help to track progress and maintain motivation.

Meal prep: Meal prepping can save time and make healthy eating more convenient. Plan meals in advance and prepare healthy snacks to prevent unhealthy choices.

Make exercise fun: Find activities that are enjoyable and incorporate them into a regular exercise routine. This can include walking, swimming, dancing, or yoga.

Practice stress management: Practice stress management techniques such as meditation, deep breathing, or yoga. Identify sources of stress and take steps to minimize them.

Get adequate sleep: Establish a regular sleep schedule and create a relaxing bedtime routine. Avoid caffeine and electronics before bedtime.

Avoid tobacco and excessive alcohol consumption: Avoid tobacco use and limit alcohol consumption to moderate levels.

Build and maintain relationships: Build and maintain relationships with family and friends. Join a social group or participate in community events.

Practice self-care: Practice self-care by engaging in activities that promote relaxation and reduce stress. This can include reading, taking a bath, or listening to music.

CHAPTER #3

HEALTHY LIFESTYLE

Overall, maintaining a healthy lifestyle involves making choices that promote good physical and mental health. By focusing on healthy eating, regular exercise, high-quality sleep, stress management, avoidance of substance use, healthy relationships, and self-care, you can promote good health and well-being.

1) Maintaining Healthy Lifestyle

1.   **Eat a balanced diet:** A healthy diet should include a variety of fruits, vegetables, whole grains, lean protein, and healthy fats. Try to limit processed foods, sugary drinks, and excessive amounts of saturated and trans fats. A healthy diet is essential for maintaining good health. Focus on consuming whole, nutrient-dense foods, such as fruits, vegetables, lean protein sources, whole grains, and healthy fats.

2.   **Stay hydrated:** Drink plenty of water throughout the day, especially when exercising or spending time in the sun. Avoid sugary drinks, energy drinks, and excessive amounts of caffeine.

3.   **Exercise regularly:** Aim for at least 30 minutes of moderate-intensity exercise most days of the week. This can include activities such as brisk walking, jogging, cycling, or swimming.

4.   Get enough sleep: Aim for 7-8 hours of sleep each night. Create a bedtime routine and stick to it, avoid using electronics before bed, and create a comfortable sleep environment.

5.   Manage stress: Practice stress management techniques such as deep breathing, meditation, or yoga. Take breaks throughout the day to stretch or go for a walk, and avoid overloading your schedule.

6.   Avoid smoking and excessive alcohol consumption: Smoking can increase the risk of cancer, heart disease, and other health problems. Excessive alcohol consumption can also increase the risk of health problems such as liver disease and cancer.

7.   Stay connected with others: Social connections can help reduce stress and improve mental health. Make time for friends and family, and participate in social activities that you enjoy.

8.   Take care of your mental health: Prioritize your mental health by practicing self-care, seeking professional help if needed, and creating a support system of friends and family.

Remember that small changes in daily habits can g overall health and well-being.

9.   Engage in regular physical activity: Regular exercise is important for maintaining good physical health, reducing the risk of chronic diseases, and improving mental health outcomes. Aim for at least 150 minutes of moderate-intensity exercise per week.

10.   Get enough high-quality sleep: Getting enough sleep is essential for good health. Aim for 7-8 hours of sleep per night, and establish a regular sleep routine to help promote high-quality sleep.

11.   Manage stress: Chronic stress can have negative effects on physical and mental health. Identify healthy ways to manage stress, such as exercise, meditation, deep breathing, or spending time in nature.

12.   Avoid substance use: Substance use, including tobacco, alcohol, and drugs, can have significant negative effects on health.

Avoiding substance use or seeking help if you struggle with addiction is important for maintaining good health.

13.   Maintain healthy relationships: Positive relationships with friends, family, and other loved ones can provide emotional support, motivation, and healthy coping mechanisms, all of which can promote good health and well-being.

14.   Practice self-care: Taking care of yourself is essential for good health. Make time for activities that bring you joy and relaxation, such as reading, taking a bath, or spending time with loved ones.

2) Various Aspects of a Healthy Lifestyle:

Furthermore to cover various aspects of a healthy lifestyle:

1.   Nutrition: Eating a healthy and balanced diet is key to maintaining good health. This chapter can cover topics such as the benefits of a diet rich in fruits, vegetables, whole grains, and lean protein, how to manage portion sizes, and how to read food labels.

2.   Physical activity: Regular exercise can help maintain a healthy weight, improve cardiovascular health, and reduce the risk of chronic diseases. This chapter can discuss the different types of physical activity, how to set realistic fitness goals, and how to find activities that are enjoyable and sustainable.

3.   Sleep: Getting enough high-quality sleep is important for overall health and well-being. This chapter can cover topics such as how much sleep is needed, how to create a sleep-conducive environment, and how to develop healthy sleep habits.

4.   Stress management: Chronic stress can have negative effects on both physical and mental health. This chapter can explore different techniques for managing stress, such as mindfulness meditation, deep breathing, and exercise.

5.   Mental health: Good mental health is crucial for overall well-being. This chapter can cover topics such as the benefits of positive thinking, how to cope with anxiety and depression, and how to build a support network of friends and family.

6.   Substance use: Excessive alcohol use and tobacco use can lead to a range of health problems. This chapter can explore the health risks associated with substance use, as well as strategies for quitting smoking or cutting back on alcohol.

7.   Environmental factors: The environment can have a significant impact on health. This chapter can cover topics such as air pollution, access to green spaces, and the importance of reducing waste and conserving resources.

8.   Relationships: Social connections are important for overall well-being. This chapter can explore the benefits of healthy relationships and the negative effects of social isolation.

9.   Preventive care: Regular health checkups and screenings can help detect health problems early and prevent chronic disease. This chapter can cover the recommended preventive care for different age groups and risk factors.

10.   Self-care: Taking care of oneself is essential for good health. This chapter can explore the benefits of self-care practices such as mindfulness, hobbies and leisure activities, and spending time in nature.

3) Healthy Diets

There are many healthy diets that have been researched and found to have numerous health benefits. Here are 10 of the best healthy diets:

1.   Mediterranean diet: This diet is rich in fruits, vegetables, whole grains, fish, nuts, and healthy fats like olive oil. It has been associated with a reduced risk of heart disease, stroke, and some cancers.

2.   **DASH diet:** This diet is designed to reduce blood pressure and focuses on whole grains, fruits, vegetables, low-fat dairy, lean protein, and healthy fats. It has been shown to lower blood pressure and improve cholesterol levels.

3.   **Vegetarian diet:** A vegetarian diet is focused on plant-based foods and can include dairy and eggs. It has been associated with a lower risk of heart disease, diabetes, and some cancers.

4.   **Vegan diet:** A vegan diet excludes all animal products, including dairy and eggs. It has been associated with a lower risk of heart disease, high blood pressure, and diabetes.

5.   **Flexitarian diet:** This diet is a primarily plant-based diet with occasional consumption of meat and animal products. It has been associated with improved heart health and weight management.

6.   **Paleolithic diet:** The paleo diet is based on the idea of eating like our ancestors, and focuses on foods that were available during the paleolithic era, such as meat, fish, fruits, and vegetables. It has been associated with weight loss and improved blood sugar control.

7.   **Whole30 diet:** The Whole30 diet is a 30-day elimination diet that removes sugar, dairy, grains, and processed foods from the diet. It has been associated with improved digestion and increased energy.

8.   **Nordic diet:** The Nordic diet is based on traditional foods from the Nordic region, and is high in fish, berries, whole grains, and vegetables. It has been associated with a reduced risk of heart disease and diabetes.

9.   **Mind diet:** The Mind diet is designed to reduce the risk of Alzheimer's disease and includes foods such as berries, leafy greens, nuts, and fish.

10.   **Ornish diet:** The Ornish diet is a low-fat, plant-based diet that emphasizes fruits, vegetables, whole grains, and legumes. It has been associated with improved heart health and weight loss.

It's important to remember that the best diet is one that you can stick to long-term and meets your individual needs and preferences. Always consult with a healthcare provider before making significant changes to your diet.

4) Healthy Habits

Here are 10 healthy habits that can help improve overall health and well-being:

1.   **Eating a balanced diet:** A healthy diet that is rich in fruits, vegetables, whole grains, lean protein, and healthy fats can provide the body with the nutrients it needs to function properly.

2.   **Drinking plenty of water:** Staying hydrated is essential for good health. Drinking plenty of water can help to improve digestion, regulate body temperature, and support healthy skin.

3.   **Exercising regularly:** Regular physical activity can help to improve cardiovascular health, maintain a healthy weight, and reduce the risk of chronic diseases such as diabetes and heart disease.

4.   **Getting enough sleep:** Getting enough high-quality sleep is important for overall health and well-being. Adults generally need 7-9 hours of sleep per night.

5.   **Managing stress:** Chronic stress can have negative effects on both physical and mental health. It's important to develop healthy coping mechanisms such as exercise, meditation, or spending time with loved ones.

6.   Practicing good hygiene: Practicing good hygiene, such as washing hands regularly, can help to prevent the spread of illness and infection.

7.   Avoiding smoking and excessive alcohol consumption: Smoking and excessive alcohol consumption are associated with a range of health problems. Quitting smoking and reducing alcohol intake can help to improve overall health.

8.   Keeping up with routine medical check-ups and screenings: Regular medical check-ups and screenings can help to detect health problems early and prevent chronic diseases.

9.   Maintaining a positive attitude: Maintaining a positive attitude can help to improve mental health and overall well-being. Engaging in activities that bring joy and practicing gratitude can help to foster a positive outlook.

10.   Connecting with others: Social connections are important for overall well-being. Connecting with others through social activities, volunteering, or spending time with loved ones can help to improve mental health and reduce feelings of loneliness.

CHAPTERS # 4

FACTORS THAT CAN AFFECT HEALTHY LIFESTYLE

1) Factors affecting

There are many factors that can affect a person's ability to maintain a healthy lifestyle. Here are some of the most important factors:

1. **Environment:** The physical and social environment in which a person lives can have a significant impact on their ability to maintain a healthy lifestyle. For example, access to healthy foods and safe places to exercise can make it easier to maintain a healthy diet and get regular physical activity.

2. **Socioeconomic status:** People with lower socioeconomic status may have less access to healthy foods and safe places to exercise, which can make it more difficult to maintain a healthy lifestyle.

3. **Genetics:** Genetic factors can play a role in a person's susceptibility to certain health conditions, such as obesity, diabetes, and heart disease.

4. **Personal beliefs and attitudes:** A person's personal beliefs and attitudes can affect their motivation to maintain a healthy lifestyle. For example, a person who believes that they have little

control over their health may be less likely to engage in healthy behaviors.

5.   **Social support:** Social support from friends and family can play a critical role in helping people maintain a healthy lifestyle. Supportive relationships can provide encouragement, accountability, and motivation to make healthy choices.

6.   **Knowledge and education:** Knowledge and education about healthy lifestyles can help people make informed decisions about their health. People with more education and knowledge about healthy lifestyles may be more likely to engage in healthy behaviors.

7.   **Stress:** Chronic stress can have negative effects on physical and mental health, and can make it more difficult to maintain a healthy lifestyle.

8.   **Work and lifestyle demands:** Busy work and lifestyle demands can make it more difficult to maintain a healthy lifestyle. For example, long work hours can make it more challenging to find time for exercise and meal preparation.

Understanding these factors can help people to identify barriers to maintaining a healthy lifestyle and develop strategies to overcome them.

2) Lifestyle choices that can affect

Health and lifestyle are closely interconnected, as the choices we make in our daily lives can have a significant impact on our overall health and well-being. Here are some ways in which lifestyle choices can affect health:

1.   **Diet:** The foods we eat can have a significant impact on our health, with a healthy diet being linked to reduced risk of chronic diseases such as heart disease, diabetes, and some cancers.

2.   **Exercise:** Regular physical activity can improve physical health outcomes such as cardiovascular health, muscle strength,

and bone density, as well as improve mental health outcomes such as reduced anxiety and depression symptoms.

3. **Sleep:** Getting enough high-quality sleep is important for overall health and well-being. Chronic sleep deprivation has been linked to an increased risk of obesity, diabetes, heart disease, and other health problems.

4. **Stress:** Chronic stress can have negative effects on physical and mental health, increasing the risk of chronic diseases, such as heart disease and depression.

5. **Substance use:** Substance use, including tobacco, alcohol, and drugs, can have significant negative effects on health, increasing the risk of a wide range of health problems, including cancer, heart disease, and liver disease.

Overall, lifestyle choices can have a significant impact on health outcomes. Adopting healthy lifestyle behaviors, such as eating a healthy diet, engaging in regular physical activity, getting enough high-quality sleep, managing stress, and avoiding substance use, can help to reduce the risk of chronic diseases and promote overall health and well-being.

CHAPTER # 5

HEALTH IMPACT ON RELATIONSHIP

1) Importance of Relationship

Relationships are an essential aspect of daily life, and they play an important role in shaping our overall well-being. Here are some reasons why relationships are important:

1. **Emotional support:** Relationships can provide emotional support during difficult times. Having someone to talk to and share experiences with can help reduce feelings of stress, anxiety, and depression.

2. **Sense of belonging:** Relationships can provide a sense of belonging and connection to others. Feeling like we are a part of a community or group can give us a sense of purpose and identity.

3. **Improved physical health:** Good relationships have been linked to better physical health outcomes, including reduced risk of chronic diseases such as heart disease and dementia.

4. **Improved mental health:** Positive relationships can improve mental health outcomes, such as reduced anxiety and depression symptoms.

5. **Increased happiness:** Strong relationships can increase feelings of happiness and satisfaction in life.

6. **Personal growth:** Relationships can also help us grow and develop as individuals. Our interactions with others can expose us to new ideas and perspectives, and help us learn new skills.

7. **Social support:** Relationships can provide social support that can help us cope with life stressors and challenges.

Overall, relationships are important for maintaining good physical and mental health, and for providing emotional support and a sense of belonging. It's important to invest time and effort in building and maintaining positive relationships with others.

2) Affects on Relationships

Relationships can have a significant impact on a person's ability to maintain a healthy lifestyle. Here are some ways in which relationships can affect healthy living:

1. **Emotional support:** Positive relationships can provide emotional support during times of stress, which can help to reduce stress and anxiety levels. This, in turn, can improve overall mental and physical health outcomes.

2. **Motivation:** Relationships can provide motivation and accountability for maintaining healthy habits, such as exercising regularly or eating a healthy diet. For example, having a workout partner can provide motivation to stick to an exercise routine.

3. **Healthy role models:** Positive relationships with people who practice healthy habits can serve as healthy role models and help to promote healthy living.

4.	**Social support:** Relationships can provide social support that can help a person cope with life stressors and challenges, which can improve overall well-being.

5.	**Healthy communication:** Positive relationships are built on healthy communication, which can help to reduce misunderstandings and conflicts that can contribute to stress and affect healthy living.

6.	**Healthy coping mechanisms:** Positive relationships can help to develop healthy coping mechanisms to deal with stress, such as spending time with friends, engaging in physical activity, or seeking support from loved ones.

Overall, positive relationships can have a significant impact on a person's ability to maintain a healthy lifestyle. Building and maintaining healthy relationships with others can provide emotional support, motivation, healthy role models, and healthy coping mechanisms, all of which can contribute to better physical and mental health outcomes.

3) Avoiding Toxic Relationship

Avoiding toxic relationships is an important aspect of maintaining good mental and emotional health. Here are some signs of a toxic relationship to watch out for:

1.	**Lack of respect:** In a toxic relationship, one or both partners may not show respect towards each other, belittle or criticize each other, or put each other down.

2.	**Controlling behavior:** A toxic partner may try to control the other partner's behavior, such as by monitoring their activities, restricting their social interactions, or making decisions without their input.

3.	**Emotional manipulation:** In a toxic relationship, one partner may use emotional manipulation to control or influence the other partner's behavior. This can include guilt-tripping, gaslighting, or using emotional outbursts to get their way.

4.   Dishonesty: Dishonesty and lack of trust are common features of toxic relationships, with one or both partners lying or hiding information from each other.

5.   Lack of communication: Communication is essential in any healthy relationship. In a toxic relationship, one or both partners may avoid communicating honestly or openly, leading to misunderstandings and conflicts.

6.   Lack of support: In a healthy relationship, partners support each other through difficult times. In a toxic relationship, one partner may be unsupportive or dismissive of the other partner's needs or feelings.

If you notice these signs in a relationship, it may be a toxic relationship. It is important to set boundaries and seek help if needed to end the toxic relationship and prioritize your mental and emotional well-being.

CHAPTER # 6

MAINTAINING HEALTHY ENVIRONMENT

Maintaining a healthy environment at home is important for promoting good health and well-being. Here are some things you can do to maintain a healthy environment at home:

1.   **Keep your home clean:** Regularly cleaning your home can help to remove dirt, dust, and other allergens that can impact indoor air quality and trigger allergies or asthma symptoms.

2.   **Use natural cleaning products:** Many commercial cleaning products contain harsh chemicals that can impact indoor air quality and contribute to health problems. Consider using natural cleaning products that are free of toxic chemicals.

3.   **Maintain proper ventilation:** Good ventilation is important for maintaining good indoor air quality. Make sure your home is well-ventilated by opening windows and doors, using exhaust fans, and investing in air purifiers if necessary.

4.   **Control moisture levels:** Excess moisture in the home can contribute to mold growth and impact indoor air quality. Keep

moisture levels under control by fixing any leaks or water damage promptly, using dehumidifiers if necessary, and maintaining proper ventilation.

5.   **Avoid smoking indoors:** Smoking indoors can impact indoor air quality and contribute to health problems such as asthma, allergies, and lung cancer. If you or anyone in your household smokes, make sure to do so outdoors.

6.   **Use natural pest control methods:** Many commercial pest control products contain toxic chemicals that can impact indoor air quality and contribute to health problems. Consider using natural pest control methods that are safe for humans and pets.

7.   **Use plants to improve indoor air quality:** Many indoor plants can help to improve indoor air quality by removing pollutants such as formaldehyde, benzene, and trichloroethylene from the air.

By following these tips, you can create a healthy environment at home that promotes good health and well-being.

CHAPTER # 7

DAILY EXERCISES TO STAY HEALTHY

Daily exercise is an important component of a healthy lifestyle. Here are some exercises that you can do daily to improve your health:

1. **Cardiovascular exercises:** Cardiovascular exercises such as running, brisk walking, cycling, swimming, and dancing are great for improving your heart health and burning calories.

2. **Strength training exercises:** Strength training exercises such as push-ups, squats, lunges, and weightlifting can help to build and tone muscles, improve bone density, and boost metabolism.

3. **Yoga:** Yoga is a great way to improve flexibility, balance, and posture. It can also help to reduce stress and promote relaxation.

4. **Pilates:** Pilates is another great way to improve flexibility, posture, and core strength. It can also help to reduce back pain and improve balance.

5. **High-intensity interval training (HIIT):** HIIT workouts involve alternating periods of high-intensity exercise with periods of rest or low-intensity exercise. They can be a great

way to burn calories, improve cardiovascular fitness, and boost metabolism.

6.   **Walking:** Walking is a simple and effective way to improve cardiovascular fitness, burn calories, and improve overall health. It's also a low-impact exercise that can be done anywhere.

7.   **Stretching:** Stretching is important for maintaining flexibility, reducing muscle tension, and improving range of motion. It can also help to reduce the risk of injury during exercise.

Remember to consult with your doctor before starting any exercise program, especially if you have any health conditions or concerns. Start with a few minutes of exercise each day and gradually increase the duration and intensity as your fitness level improves. Aim for at least 30 minutes of moderate-intensity exercise most days of the week for optimal health benefits.

Good Bye......!

A big Thank You for reading it and reached here!!
I wish you the best of your health, may you get what you want for and keep reading my books for more healthy content........
My prayers are always with you all.